# THE TRUTH ABOUT
# THE TRUTH

# JAHRED RICE

**ISBN-13:** 978-1-7341797-5-0

**Library of Congress Control Number**: 2020904811

Published by LaBoo Publishing Enterprise
Cover photography by Jeffrey Rice, Jr.
Cover design by Navi Roberts

For information regarding special discounts for bulk purchases, please contact the publisher: LaBoo Publishing Enterprise, LLC
staff@laboopublishing.com
www.laboopublishing.com

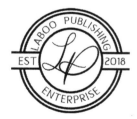

Printed in the United States of America
Baltimore, Maryland

# DEDICATION

This book is dedicated to my late friend, Keshon Nowlin; an amazing, loving, strong and courageous man, son and friend. #LongLiveKeshon

# ACKNOWLEDGEMENTS

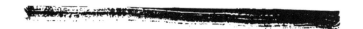

I want to thank from the bottom of my heart the people who have helped in the journey of writing this book. To my amazing mother Kimmoly LaBoo, my brother Jeffrey Rice, Jr., Kaylin Cabble, Joshua Carr, Rukiya McCormick, and Fresh Redding; thank you for all the big parts you've played, not only in this book, but in my life. I love you all dearly.

# TABLE OF CONTENTS

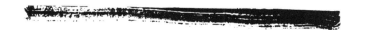

# INTRODUCTION

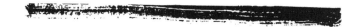

"Great morning, Jahred Rice!" Many have heard this phrase leave my mouth, and if you have and are reading this now, I'd like to think you probably chuckled as you read it in my voice. This one statement is not only a mantra that I used every day in college, but one I use every day and in every aspect of my life. To the surprise of many, the phrase did not start with me. I first heard "Great morning!" from a friend of mine, during my senior year of high school in our English class. We had a teacher who every morning, the first class of the day, would sing "good morning" everyone. She was this small, short in stature, sweet-hearted older lady. Each day she would start the class by taking attendance, and after calling each name she'd look up at you and say, "Good morning!" My friend had transferred into our school and our class about midway through the school year, and he was the type of guy that you knew he was present. When he walked in a room you knew he was there. As our teacher went through student after student, we would all reluctantly reply, with sleep in our eyes and mouth, "Good morning," many not even looking up at her as we said it. We all waited in expectation for my friend's turn though. We knew what would come out of his mouth every time. Our teacher would call his name and before she could even finish her "Good morning" he'd chant back, with authority in his voice and projection, "GREAT MORNING!" One day our teacher asked him why he'd say that, and his answer was that, every day he woke up, was able to eat and had clothes on his back, so how is it not a great day?

I went to a performing arts school for college, where I was quickly introduced to a slate line. Prior to coming to the school, I had no idea what "slating" was. I saw each person, one by one, essentially step out of line, introduce themselves, and then step back in. Being that my last name was Rice, I was lucky to stand at the end of each of these lines. I quickly observed two things. The first thing I noticed was that this was an opportunity for all eyes to be on you—an opportunity to have the spotlight and to stand out. The second was that everyone did and said the same exact thing. It was boring. I thought to myself, how could anyone be different or special in this type of system. I also, since I was very young, had a problem with being just like everybody else. Something about that always made my skin crawl until this day. I always heard and believed that I was extremely special and unique, so when I was basically being told or encouraged to be just like everyone else in an environment where I knew standing out couldn't possibly be frowned on, I decided to be different. When it was my turn to step out of line, I remembered my friend from high school "Great morning." I thought about his explanation and I knew right then that would be the one line that separated me and showed everybody who I was. I stepped forward confidently and boldly, and said with full projection so all could hear, "GREAT MORNING! Jahred Rice!" From that first day I continued not only to say it, it became a trademark for me as a person, and my loving, outgoing, and optimistic personality, that everyone at my school would know me for.

I live by that phrase every day of my life and I make sure to not only look at my current circumstances, no matter what they be, as great or going to be great. I choose to live a life of greatness and I choose every single day to embark on a journey to leave a legacy of greatness. I aim to leave a legacy that God would be proud of, and a legacy that not only touches hundreds of generations after me but also one that has eternal impact.

Writing this book is a part of that greatness and my legacy. I wrote this book to share my truth in hopes that it would liberate and bring revelation, healing, and the love of God to all who read it. This book is a culmination of personal short stories from my adolescence and growing up as a young brown man in Baltimore, Maryland. This book highlights some of my good times, and my bad times, from my struggles with depression, thoughts of suicide, and the topic of homosexuality, to early teenage trauma I experienced during a home invasion, and the lessons I've learned from them all.

In this book I have shared my poetry/spoken word, dreams, revelations and inner thoughts and conversations I've had with God over the past years. I pray this book will allow anyone who reads it to be encouraged to defeat fear and live in their own truth, whatever that may be. In Ephesians 4:25 it reads, "Therefore having put away falsehood let each one of you speak the truth with his neighbor for we are members of one another." I believe it is our job to use our truth to help and heal one another and that our lives are all connected, and we need each other. I pray that you understand that everything you've ever gone through can and will be used for your good and that the love of God will propel you to greater heights than you've ever imagined, and out of even the darkest of holes you could ever find yourself in. In Ephesians 3:16 it says, "And I pray that He would unveil within you the unlimited riches of His glory and favor until supernatural strength floods your innermost being with His divine might and explosive power." I pray that this book may be a vessel to bring you strength, courage, and closer to God, your truth and the truth that is Jesus and his love for you: as well as the fact that he loves you no matter the circumstance and just wants you to be in a close and intimate relationship with him.

Lastly, I want to say thank you for deciding to read this book. I believe you didn't pick it up by accident or coincidence, but because it was meant for you to read at this appointed time in your life. I know the truth shared in this book is timeless and has the eternal hand of God on it. Please, kick back and enjoy this book that is my life and my truth. I challenge you, as you read and once you've finished, to walk into your truth and have the courage to be GREAT!

# CHAPTER ONE
# THE GREEN BROWNIE
# (10ᵀᴴ GRADE)

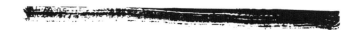

Growing up I went to two different high schools. This story is about the first high school I went to, named Milford. It was a pretty unique school, because it was a mix of three different school types. Milford was a magnet school, insofar as it was big on performing arts, singing, dancing, acting. But it was also like a regular high school you would see in the movies. You had kids who were great singers and dancers, there were kids in cosmetology, and there was even engineering magnet kids. Just like any other school, though, you had the kids who were classic troublemakers, and oftentimes I found myself in the middle of every group. The reason Milford had such a diverse population was probably due to its location. Although Milford was in a sort of rural location, it was right along Liberty Road, which runs into the city.

Now as a kid, I loved to eat. I loved snacks and anything un-healthy. My favorite thing to eat when it came to snacks was brownies. I just loved the chocolate. The texture of it is an over-all masterpiece of a food, something I definitely could never turn down. And if I could eat them for the rest of my life with no physical consequences or health issues, I would do it, no question.

I had a best friend that was from Honduras. She was light skinned, had long hair, and was a girly-girl kind of tomboy. She was edgy, sociable, and funny. She could be crude, and she may have been a compulsive liar, but she was my best friend. We pretty much did everything together. We knew everybody at our school, and we were in the in-crowd in the midst of just about everything that happened, whether it involved us or not. We knew who played sports, who was dating who, and even people who sold drugs. It was the best. Being this type of person causes you to fall into things rather unexpectedly, and these pop-ups happened on a frequent basis. So, one day everything was as it always was, ordinary, basic, unpredictable, and unusual. It was third period, and at my school the lunch periods were broken up into about three or four different sections, all taking place throughout the third period time block. This semester, my third period class was math, and my lunch was scheduled right in between that class. This meant that I would go to class for about 45 minutes, then we would have a break and go to lunch, and then come back for another 30 to 20 minutes to finish that same class.

As I got to lunch that day, I remember doing the usual – getting my food, sitting down at the same table as always – and I remember my best friend wasn't there. She would usually always be right there whenever I came in the cafeteria, so that day it was a little weird that she wasn't even in the cafeteria yet. But then again, with her being the type of person she was, always getting into something, I didn't really think anything of it, I just wondered where she was. Sure enough, about ten minutes into the lunch period she finally made her way into the cafeteria and sat down at our table. Once she sat down, I asked her where she'd been. She said, "Don't worry about it." So, what do you do when somebody says don't worry about it? Obviously you start to think about it even more and you want to know. Seconds later she pulls out this plastic bag with what looked to be four beautiful, gorgeous, mouthwatering, tongue-swelling, drool-engaging chocolate brownies. Immediately I snatched the bag out of her hand and said, "Let me get one." As it was entering my mouth, she simply said, "Ok." Now I want to pause for a second, because this was an unusual response. In general, when somebody asks you for something, you usually have a little push back. The first response we typically get is not a casual, nonchalant, "OK." So, after she didn't fight me on it, I decided to have another one.

Fast forward, and I'm back in my math class after lunch, and now is where things started to take a turn. The way our math class usually went was, before the end of every class, before you could leave, you had to finish your assignment and turn it in, and that was your ticket out of the door. I usually finished my

assignments early so I would just get up, turn it in and then re-
turn to my seat and wait for the bell to ring. When I got up to
turn in my finished assignment, I stood up quickly. Something
kind of hit me, and it was like the room spun. I got dizzy, but
then it went right away just as quick as it came. I didn't think
anything of it, and I just went and turned my paper in.

Thirty minutes later, I was in my last period of the day, gym
class. Now in gym class a lot of times if you didn't feel like par-
ticipating you just didn't dress, and you came up with whatever
excuse you needed to and usually the gym teacher wouldn't even
bat an eyelid at you. On this day I did not want to do anything,
because they were playing badminton, so me and a friend of
mine we decided that we were just going to sit on the side, which
we did. As I was sitting on the side, I started to feel the dizziness
again and this time was way more intense. Then as I was sitting
with my back against the wall, I started to feel like I was slowly
getting pulled into the wall. Now I know this may sound crazy
but I'm not making this up. I started to feel as if the wall was
pulling me in for a really tight hug or I was getting pulled into a
wall of quicksand.

That was when it all started to hit me really bad. I remember there
being a guy that was a maintenance worker with a huge ladder
in the gym fixing something in the rafters. I was so locked in
on him until my vision started to scatter. My vision became like
one of those fly vision videos on YouTube, where there's about
eight different lenses. It was like it was being thrown in circles.

I'm sure by now you've figured out that the brownies I had eaten before weren't regular brownies.

I looked over to my friend, and he began to laugh. He said, "Bro, you look smacked." When you look smacked, it's basically saying you look really, really, high. So, at this point I'm feeling it in every sense of the word. My senses felt enhanced and my reactions were delayed. I remember my friend telling some of the other guys that I was hard, and they started to punch me in my arm, but I didn't feel a thing. Yeah, I was pretty done. But that's not the end of the story.

The hardest part of being high at this point was the fact that I had a dance practice after school. I had just started dancing, so I didn't know anything about dance. I hadn't ever trained, I just did it because it was fun. But this day, out of all days, there happened to be a new routine that we had to learn. I thought, *I'll be fine, I'll be able to manage.* I went to the dressing room, splashed some water on my face and thought that I would be good. As I came out and began to watch them do the combination, it looked like the hardest dance steps I had ever seen in my life. I tried to do them, and I was so delayed and slow it was a disaster. At that point I knew there was no hope for me, so I snuck back into the dressing room, grabbed my things, and I walked out the side door without anybody even noticing.

I remember that day just walking around school with my iPod – yes, my iPod: this was in 2012 guys – just listening to Drake's song "Show me a good time" on repeat. After walking around aimlessly in circles at my school, my dad came to pick me up and of course, still high as ever, I got in the car. But instead of going home he decided to take me to get a haircut. *THIS DAY NEVER ENDS*, I thought to myself.

I remember sitting in the barber's chair, the room still spinning, but at this point I was slumped. I was dozing off in the chair and could barely keep my head up. I had to keep picking my head up, it was terrible. When I got home that night I went straight to sleep, knocked out cold. Now why did I choose to share this story? I guess to teach a simple lesson: you should not always eat home goods that aren't from your home.

# CHAPTER TWO
# DOORS

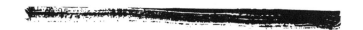

## Part 1

Most people who know me now would say I'm outgoing, goofy, outspoken, loud, animated, fearless and always looking on the bright side or having a great attitude regarding life. These are all things I've heard people say about me when I asked them to describe me. All these things are true, and all these things were always a part of me and who I am. But there was a time where these traits were suppressed and definitely not the way I saw myself. I believe I am the way I am now because of what I've been through and my ability, through God's strength, to use it as my "why" in life. I decided that since I've been through the darkness, I know what's there, so I should be the light that illuminates it. Since I've been in the bottom of the pit, I should be the rope others can use to climb out of it.

Around the time I was about 12 or 13, my mom got remarried and she, me, my brother, and my then-stepdad moved into a new, big house in a nice, quiet suburban community in Maryland. This house would be where I spent most of my adolescence and where a lot of who I am today was shaped, good and bad. Under this one roof I learned so much about life, love, relationships, sex, trauma, and much more. I lived there until I was about 16, but in those short years a lot happened. I experienced my mother endure a toxic relationship of verbal abuse, and witnessed aggressions from my stepdad that, in hindsight, had effects on me up until this day.

In this house there were three levels: an upstairs; a main floor that included the living room, dining room and kitchen; and a basement. For basically the entirety of my time there I remember my house being split up. As a family we lived under the same roof, but we were about as separate as if we'd lived in houses across a state line. My mom spent a lot of time in her office room, which was on the second floor (upstairs). My stepdad spent all his time in the basement, even sleeping there most of the time. I frequented the living room, where the TV with cable was, and my brother's room, which was home for the video game.

As time passed in this house, I began to experience the strain of my mom's struggling marriage right before my eyes. My stepdad had a real mean streak and an awful temper. He would often get agitated and annoyed with the smallest of things: you accidentally eating or drinking the last of something that in his head he deemed as solely belonging to him, to being upset because he had to wait an extra two minutes in the car while we were rushing to leave to go somewhere. I do not know the full extent of the issues my mom and he faced within their marriage, but I do know his actions and reactions to whatever may have been going on did impact me traumatically.

One thing he often did that I've noticed still has an effect on me is the way he'd express his frustration. His main go to when he was angry or upset would be to stomp very loudly down every single step, and there were two doors that led down to the basement that he would slam extremely hard on his way down there. I noticed that experiencing that has had a lasting impact on me. Now, no matter where I'm at – school, home, anywhere – if a door slams, my mind immediately jumps to the memories of growing up in those situations. A flashback automatically triggered, and my body tenses up briefly before I tell myself that there is no threat of harm and I can allow myself to relax.

In college I lived in four different dorm rooms. The fourth room I lived in had a really heavy door and it would pretty much slam closed every time you went in and out if you didn't hold on to it as it closed. There would be times at night where I'd be sleeping and in the middle of the night my roommate would either come in or go out and mistakenly let the door slam, and it would make me jump out of my sleep. I'd shoot open my eyes on high alert and for a split second there I was, back in that house I grew up in. As a kid you don't really realize the lasting effects some things will have on you, but as an adult I see them now, and I hope that anyone reading this will be extremely cautious about what you do or allow children and teens to experience.

It was during my time in that house that I began to experience my stint of depression and self-harm. I'd be a fool to say that the things my stepdad put my mom and myself through didn't, in part, contribute to that. I'm not saying it was the bottom-line reason for my depression, but it definitely played a part in it. I witnessed unhealthy ways of coping with emotions and feelings, which led me to deal with my emotions the only way I had been subliminally taught, which was unhealthily.

* * * * * *

## Part 2

In middle school there were several things I can remember that caused me to have a skewed vision and perception of my-self. I was a bit chubby in middle school and I remember being ashamed of it and wondering why I wasn't skinny like some other kids I hung out with. I also was a bit jealous of all the nice clothes that other kids had. They'd have on all these expensive name brands that I never had because my mom would never spend her money on expensive clothes for no reason. Now this is not to say that I had beat up clothes or anything, they just weren't what the "cool kids" had, and so not being a part of that crowd also made me question my own self-value.

I distinctly remember a long period of time where I felt that I had no friends whatsoever. I had a Spanish class in eighth grade with a few people who were, like me, sort of class clowns. In that class the desks were set up as tables, and there were only four seats to a table. There were five of us class clowns in that class, so if you do the math, one person was the odd man out every class. Most times it was whichever of us got into class last that wouldn't make the cut. Usually I'd make it to the table and be fine, but there were some times I wouldn't. I don't know why, but when I didn't sit with them, my little heart and ego was bruised.

Now as kids we really had no filter on what came out of our mouths most times. Being the clowns, most days, whoever didn't make it to the table, we would pick on and crack jokes about them for the duration of the class. Usually it didn't bother me too much. I'd usually clap back with my own jokes from across the room. But one day in particular, I sort of came to a point where I couldn't take it. On this day, I had a fight with my girlfriend, and that had me in my feelings.

I went into Spanish class this day and I didn't make the table. As I sat at the other table essentially alone, I could hear the other kids snickering and see them looking my way and then laughing. Now that I was already upset from the events prior, I started to feel extremely alone and ostracized. I had bit of a mental breakdown and couldn't take it anymore. This overwhelming anger and sadness came over me, and I got up and stormed out of the classroom. That same night was the first night I ever cut myself. I was in my room and I turned off all the lights. I hated everything about myself all of a sudden. I felt ugly, fat, and unwanted. So I went in the closet in my room and I grabbed my big winter bubble coat. I put on many layers of clothes and the coat over top, thinking that would somehow make me lose weight. I went into the closet and sat in the corner and closed the door behind me, so it was completely pitch-black dark. I sat in there for about ten minutes crying and quietly swearing at myself, and all the events of the day were replaying over and over in my head.

I cried until there were no more tears to cry. I began to feel numb, as if I had just cried out all my emotions. I then got up and went back out into my room. Now this is the part where I can directly connect the trauma with my stepdad to me harming myself. Because my stepdad often made me feel extremely unsafe, I would hide knives all throughout the house, including in my room. The fear he made me feel caused me to think that one day I would need to protect me and my mom from him. Getting back to that night, I recalled that I had hid a knife under my bed. I got the knife and sat on my bed. I took off all the clothes I had on and I began to cut up and down the inside of my left arm. That night I cut myself five times, one after the other, trying to see how deep I could go. It was this weird sense of release when I did it, and in that moment that was all I wanted. I had been holding in so much that I wanted to let it go, and that's the only way I knew how.

I was first introduced to cutting in eighth grade by my friend, who was like my best friend/girlfriend. We always sat next to each other in the classes we had together, and I would see her arm and she had scars all up and down them. I asked her what they were from and she told me she did them to herself. Me being young and dumb, I remember thinking it looked sort of cool. One day she came to class and she had a scar, but this one was way different than the rest. She had cut the word HATE into her arm. She that day explained that she didn't cut for fun, but to escape what she was feeling. After the first time I cut, I knew what she'd been talking about. After that first time I started to do it more and more often, so much so, I couldn't even tell you a concrete number of how many times I had. Pretty much all my scars have healed to the point of no visibility, but if I look at my arm and think of that time in my life, I can see them clear as day. Another moment of my life I remember as clear as day is when I fell victim to a home invasion/robbery.

• • • • • •

## Part 3

The biggest hit to my ego was when I was the victim of a home invasion. I use the word "ego" because I believe the word means that what everyone else thinks of you goes. It was the end of the school day, on a day towards the end of the school year. We were allowed to go outside for a lot of our classes. I was with a girl who was my friend at the time. We hung out a lot inside and outside of school. She introduced me to sex, drugs, and hanging out with older people. Anytime we hung out, we were doing one of those things.

This day was supposed to be no different. When we were outside, she asked if I knew whether my parents would be home. I told her they should be, and that she could come over and we would hang out. Later that day we rode the bus home from school and as we got off the bus, I told her to just come and ring my doorbell when she was ready for me to come out. After some time passed, I went to sit on my front step and waited for her to come over. Another girl that lived with her came from around the corner up to the doorstep of my house and asked if it was okay for my friend to come over now. I said yes, and she went away.

About two minutes later a guy that I'd never seen before began to walk out in front of the house. At first, he walked past the house, and then doubled back and asked if I had a phone that he could use. Now usually I am very on guard and hesitant when it comes to people in general. This time was no different, but I decided to stop being so paranoid and just try to do a good thing. So, I decided to say yes, and I walked in to get the house phone from inside of the house. I walked back and gave him the phone. I noticed that he was dialing numbers but never really connecting with anyone. At that moment I figured out what was going on. He told me to get up and go into the house. I wasn't shocked by what he said, because I had already put two and two together.

When we got in the house he asked if anyone was there, and I said no. He told me to get on the floor. At first, I resisted, then he got aggravated and so he forced me down to the floor. Then he was on top of me and at this point I didn't know what he was going to do, so I started to struggle and fight back. I hit him in his face once, and then he punched me several times. I kept scooting back, trying to get away. We struggled for about thirty seconds throughout the dining room, until he picked up a magazine rack and hit me in my head with it twice. At that point I stopped struggling. He told me to turn onto my stomach, and he made me put my hands behind my back and zip-tied them. After that he made me stand up, and then he told me to take him to the rooms that had stuff that he could take.

He held onto my arm and made me walk up the steps to the top floor and went from bedroom to bedroom. He made me sit on the floor while he ransacked the place looking for things he could take. After he was done with all the rooms upstairs, he then took me to the basement where my stepdad had all his valuable possessions. In the basement we went into his music room where he kept most of his watches that he valued a lot. As he began to take the watches and put them in his bag at that moment, I had a thought. I thought I could lock him in the room and run. But I wasn't sure if he had other people with him, so I decided not to try it.

Then he walked me into the basement storage room. He then told me to face away from him and lay down. At this moment I remember talking to God. I asked Him to not let him kill me... then I remember thinking at the same time, if it was my time to go, I would be okay with it. I think I've always kind of had that realization that when it is time, it is time. The older I get the less and less afraid of death I am because ultimately, I know where I am going. I think back to Pastor Tim Ross talking about his aunt that was diagnosed with cancer, and before one of her surgeries they were all upset, and she said to them that one of two things would happen: either God would heal her of her sickness and they would give him all the glory, or he wouldn't and she would be in Glory. Ever since I heard that story, the fear of dying doesn't really hit me as hard as it used to. I still don't want to die – I don't think anybody really does – but I am not paralyzed by the fear of death. Eventually the robber ran out through the basement door and disappeared.

After that incident happened, I was in the hospital for a day with a bunch of scars, bruises and broken braces, etc. In the coming days we found out that the friend who I often hung out with was the mastermind behind it all. She set the whole thing up. She knew the guy and they planned to rob me. That feeling of betrayal really hurt a lot.

After the incident, I stayed at my dad's house. Most of the time I spent there was in the basement where I played video games. On one occasion, I went to use the bathroom. As I went to wash my hands, I looked at myself in the mirror and I saw how my face was all bruised and swollen. I literally broke down in tears and I hated what I saw. I didn't even recognize who I was. The swelling was bad, and I just hated it. Mixed with all the lingering self-doubt and depression months before the incident even happened, this was when I fell into my darkest and deepest hole. I felt betrayed by one of my closest friends and I felt lonelier than I had before because I wasn't going to school. I kept replaying the incident over and over and wondering what I could have done differently: if I could have fought back more, hadn't been so naïve, or hadn't went to get him the phone.

But through my time off, somehow God was able to penetrate the darkness that I was in and I started to think about everyone that was affected by this and not just myself. I thought about my mom, my dad, my brother, the guy that did it. Still till this day I can't really explain how or why, but I began to come to terms with it all and started to feel this sense of empathy and compassion for everyone involved.

I think I realized that day that I could have lost my life, but I realized that since I didn't, me being angry and negative was not the right response to me being able to live another day. I started to really recognize all that God had done for me and what he was to me, which was love. I knew that I needed to share that with the people that needed that the most, which was the guy and the girl that had done this to me. I decided to forgive them, and ever since that situation, day by day, up until now, I have taken a step towards love, towards compassion, wholeness, peace and joy.

Speaking on all these situations and incidents that led me to my period of depression, I can't help but also think that these were the things that are ultimately leading me to my greatness as well. As I look back on all these events, I realize that through all of them God was always with me, replenishing the love that was taken from me, restoring the peace the enemy tried to steal from me, and overflowing me with joy, enough for me to share with everyone I've come to know. Even now as I am writing these stories about what I have been through and what I have overcome, I feel a new sense of healing taking place. I've talked about all these situations with several people before but writing it all out is a healing you can't hide from. Seeing these words on the page and not just as words that disappear as I say them has caused me to really face them and ask myself whether I have really dealt with them and healed from them.

I want to encourage everyone who reads this to be bold and courageous enough to write down what you have been through if you can. I know it's not an easy task but doing so may help you to heal like it has helped me. I know and understand that depression is a real thing and it is easy to go at it alone, but I also wish that anyone dealing with it would be brave enough to ask for help. Know that it is a hole that you can climb out of, and it does not dictate who you will be. What you have been through, good or bad, is an opportunity. Use it to push you to who you are called to be.

The following outlines a process you can use to do this.

# FIVE STEPS TO
# TURNING TRAUMA INTO TRIUMPH

## Acknowledge Your Hurt, Pain and Shame

In order to really heal anything, we must first know what the problem is as well as the severity of the problem. If we fail to realize a problem exists, then we can't possibly hope to heal and become a better person.

## Trace Your Pain

This is certainly a lot easier said than done. We must be brave enough to see clearly the root from which our negative behavior stems. Once you identify the person or situation that hurt you, you have the ability to forgive. An example in my story is the anxiousness and anger I would feel when people would walk too closely behind me in public places. I would get really upset about it, until one day a friend of mine asked me why. I had never really thought of that; I just assumed everyone would be bad. I then started to realize that I wasn't just feeling uncomfortable. I would let that small of a thing control my entire energy for some time, which was extremely unhealthy. I did some tracing that night and I finally put two and two together and figured out where this all came from. When I was betrayed by my friends and robbed in middle school, that experience robbed me of my sense of security and had me believing everyone was always up to something, always trying to harm me in some way. This realization leads me to number three.

## Know Your Triggers

It is important to be aware of the situations you are in and the people you are surrounded by, and to notice what triggers past traumas to arise. Pay attention to what makes you think of that tough time. Also remain aware of how you are responding in these situations, and your thoughts too.

As I stated before, one of my triggers came when people I didn't know came too close to me. Know your triggers so you stop pulling them on innocent people.

## Change Your Response

Now that you know you have pain, where your pain comes from, what makes your trauma kick in and the ways it makes you react, it's time to make a change.

From now on the answer is simple: be aware of yourself in all situations and refuse to let your pain, fear and emotions get the better of you. YOU CONTROL THEM, NOT THE OTHER WAY AROUND.

## Share Your Story

This may be the MOST IMPORTANT STEP! You must share your story.

One of the biggest reasons people can't overcome their struggles and trauma is because they believe that they are all alone in what they are dealing with and that nobody understands.

Your story has the power to liberate other people who are going through what you've already conquered.

This also builds community. We as humans long for a sense of people and belonging. Having a community of people who "get it" can make all the difference.

# CHAPTER THREE
# DREAMS

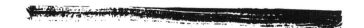

This section is a culmination of several dreams that I believe to be very prophetic and meaningful. All these dreams came to me at different points in my life, mostly when I had spent a good amount of time either meditating or being with God directly prior to going to sleep. I encourage you to always try to remember your dreams, write them out and try to find meaning in them. Dreams are one of the many ways God can speak to you, so never negate the value of dreams.

● ● ● ● ● ●

## Dream 1 (2017)

This was the last day before the end of the world. Everyone was very anxious. Everyone felt what was happening but couldn't quite understand. Then a huge bright light shone and blinded us all, and there was a building-up sound, like an earthquake. Then my neck snapped, but it didn't hurt after I was transferred and taken into the immediate presence of God. I was on my way to him. I was approaching his throne, and I was so filled with joy and I simply said, "I love you God."

• • • • • •

## Dream 2 (2017)

I was in a small room with Bishop T. D. Jakes and one other man who I believe was either Pastor Touré Roberts or Devon Franklin. We were sitting there, and the presence of the Lord was there with us. I began to speak as the Holy Spirit led and I reached out as I was praying and touched the forehead of Touré. With that touch I felt the Spirit of God move and increase in me. Then, as I reached to touch Bishop Jakes, he quickly touched my head, and a fire of God in the Holy Spirit completely took over my entire being. I began to speak in tongues so loudly and with so much conviction. I also let out yells and groans at the top of my voice, extremely loud.

I believe this dream was God anointing me to be a pastor. I also think this dream was to awaken me and make me aware that there is a huge fire on the inside of me that God is pulling out of me. I receive it Jesus. I receive it in Jesus' name. Amen

• • • • • •

## Dream 3 (2018)

I was in my room and outside my window I could see this city far off, and there was a body of water surrounding it. I watched a huge plane literally fall out of the sky and crash into the water by the city, and I knew it was the end times. I felt God tell me that. Then I wound up outside in this city and people were panicking but also trying to live ignorantly, as if nothing had happened. On the news they kept saying or denying the end times and saying the plane crash was a horrible terrorist attack, but they never said there were any people on the plane. I was speaking to someone who also knew it was the end times and saying how crazy it was that they were choosing to be oblivious to what was going on.

● ● ● ● ● ●

## Dream 4 (2018)

My mom and I drove down this steep hill/road, and at the bottom was a beach filled with people. Once we got to the bottom we got out of the car. I noticed the waves of the ocean became massive and tall, and then me and my mom and almost everyone else began to run in the other direction. We wound up running up these stairs in what appeared to be a random mall, trying to escape the water as it began to flood everything. I was with my mom and a guy that I don't know and there was a broken escalator we needed to get up, so I ran and jumped up, then helped pull my mom up. Somehow the guy with us ended up dying, but his last words to us were for us to go on without him and he'd be fine. We continued on and I woke up.

• • • • • •

## Dream 5 (2018)

There was a bombing attack in New York or East Coast, and we all heard about it on the news. We were in LA. Then a loud explosion went off and these huge missile shaped things came hurtling towards us and we were in the streets and it was complete chaos. There were three or four of us we were best friends. Three missiles came and hit in the area where we were running. We just barely avoided them, but the third one hit my friend and killed him right in front of my eyes. I was devastated and heartbroken. Then the rest of my friends pushed me to keep moving to get to safety.

• • • • • •

## Dream 6 (2019)

My mom and I were on a plane about to land in what seemed like Thailand. I looked out of the plane window and I saw the ocean waves huge as buildings crashing violently. The waves were all the way up in the air, almost as high as the plane. Then I wound up getting in my mom's car with her and a city evacuation alarm went off. The parking lot began to flood, and people were running when my mom's car turned into a boat. We ended up going to this patio. When we were there, I knew this was the end times and I was going to die there. My main concern was trying to reach my girlfriend just to hear her one last time, and to make sure our family was good.

# CHAPTER FOUR
# SPOKEN WORD/POETRY

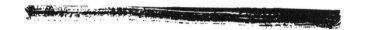

The following is a collection of poems, spoken word pieces and original song lyrics as well as song remixes. These serve as insights to my heart. This was one of the easiest ways I found to express my emotions about several heartbreaks regarding different romantic relationships going south. Let these words, rhymes, similes and versus be the antidote to a heart cauterizing the wounds of torn connections.

# ALPHA

The beginning of me is where I find my identity, created and conceptualized all in the hands of my Father. Sons and daughters, we were all thought of. And when I think about our Father all I feel is love, and there's no other version out there that could compare. I try to find it in the mirror sometimes; I just get stuck in the stare. Try to find it in my friends, ain't no love out there. I even looked between her thighs, then it all became clear: if I keep looking round this earth I ain't gon' find it nowhere. So now I'm looking to the one above, the one that thought of me, lined up my genealogy, gave me all this authority. Beginning and the end, inner and outer, Omega yea that's my Father, sometimes I may call him ALPHA.

# MY PAIN EQUALS 55

I never made a piece about love, in my experience it never fit like a glove. It was more like dirty laundry swept under the rug, and I'm so nose blind it didn't cause me to budge, and your skin was so delectable the best kind of fudge. I put my head right by your heart girl, I just wanted a hug. But when I told you that I love you all I got was a shrug. And now I'm wondering, how the hell everyone else fall in love. Now I'm sitting here, face like a pug, trying to mute romantic sorrows with all these types of drugs. Just moved a Lay-Z Boy into the hole that I dug. Man ain't it crazy tryna beat out one drug with another drug? That's what love is, and it comes with addiction, that leaves you checking phones and pressing folks that's tryna mess with your prescription. Got you listenin, got you wishing that you weren't Christian, cuz if she press up on your man then that's a wave cap missing. Now hold on, ladies I know you not the only crazy ones, cuz I then pulled a few triggers on some dialectal guns, ready to pop on any dude staring at my baby's buns, and I let everyone in the room know she ain't the one.

Shoot, this got me hot. She love me, love me not, got my stomach tied in knots. Think I need one more shot, and then I'll give it one more shot, need to shoot before the clock. Oh shoot, there she is. What do I say? I forgot. Now she all way up the block. Crazy thing is we had chemistry, I guess not. I wonder if she knows this is about her or did it go over her top? Crazy thing is I was gon' give her all that I got. Between a hard place and a rock, she walked past and didn't speak, then my stomach just dropped. Ain't heard from her in like four days and I'm thinkin' Why not, what I do wrong? Can't believe that I just blew up this spot. But hey, I guess you live and you learn. Everyone goes thru heartbreak and I guess it's my turn. I didn't know the word crush was a literal term, and she never texted back, rejection confirmed. I guess now I know why I never wrote about love: it was something I never won at, we were just playing fictional characters in a cheesy one act. If I could get back all the time, I wouldn't take it back. If I could unwrite all these rhymes, nah I wouldn't do that. Forget the inside of your thighs or the freckles on your back, my hands racing up your racetrack, and all the sounds you made when I pressed up on that... I wouldn't, cuz it meant something to me, maybe just a touch for you, but it drove me wild, mammoth, wooly...and I don't think you'll ever understand how much I loved you fully. 11, 1, 4, 25, 14, those numbers meant something like your name meant to me.

• • • • • •

# HYPATHETAFANTACLISMIC — IMPOSSIBLE INEVITABILITY

Listen to me, be understanding. I'm just asking, I'm not demanding. Want you with me when storms are crashing. My heart's been kidnapped, your love's my ransom. Listen to me, be understanding. I'm just asking, I'm not demanding. Want you with me when the storms are crashing? If I can never be your lover maybe I can be your friend. Let me say that you just started something you got me far from laughing. I can't believe you got me thinking about the thoughts of cuffin'. Am I rushin'? Might be rushin' yeah. I said I just might be rushin' but having you right by my side makes me scared of nothing.

I can't believe I found somebody that could elevate me. Got me feeling super good. Baby go and cape me.

I wanna wrap my hands around a spinal cord of your existence. When we first met you didn't really seem to spark my interest, you were persistent. A Hypathetafantaclismic closing distance friendship that was instant, but I kind of missed it. I've been feening for the comfort of your safety lately. If we came this far, why would we give it up? I wonder after all we've been through; do you hate me? Especially now, cuz you see all my flaws in HD? Nothing worse than watching tears fall from your mother's eyes. The stories are kinda sad, but men are not allowed to cry. I hope I don't go fall asleep on this here lullaby, my hood lullaby.

# DISCONNECTED

God what's your number? Cuz I'm trying to reach you, trying to learn something that these schools can't teach you. You said I could call you anytime, but most times I'm scared to hit your line. I'm ashamed of the things that I've done, and the thing I want to share never leaves my mind. I start crying, cuz I feel when I call you, you'll press decline. My mental health and wellness is damn near in decline, so complacent where I'm at my spirit is on recline, living day to day having thoughts that are mine! I tried to cry but I'm all cried out. Don't hear my name anymore, when it comes from your mouth. If you're the streams of living water, then my soul's in a drought. I can't come out, not on my own at least. Trust me, I tried, and I tried, all it got me was grief. The heaviness is weighing on me. God, I need some relief. My life is filled with so much drama, needs some comic relief before I'm deceased. And I can't blame it on the white man. The white man ain't put this blunt in my hand, the white man ain't put the blunt to my lip, tricking me into sexing a chick. Nah, the white man only did one thing, be a white man, so if you think it's his fault life isn't going to plan, then got damn, how 'bout you ask who's playing. Is it yours or is it God's? Please hear what I'm saying: I get mad at God too my brother, it's not just you. Hella nights that I cried till my face turn blue, outside cursing out the sky, thinking his promise ain't true. What do I do? Let me get back to you on that, cuz me and God ain't really cool. I'll let you know when we on track.

# MANTALITY

Man, I been around the block. Had these females on lock. I had like seven or eight between these legs like six and nine on the clock. Six foot nine? Prolly not, but Imma always shoot my shot, cuz just like Thanksgiving dinner, Imma get it while it's hot.

What? Ya'll looking at me wrong, but this the way I was brought up. Do your dirt, don't get caught up. Y'all hating the player but not the game. But these chicks I must maintain. But if she wind up on some games, then that's a game that I'm not playin'.

I never questioned who I am. I make money, got the yams. Half of that to Uncle Sam, and the broads know who I am. To sum it up all in one word, shoot I'd say that I'm the MAN. I'm the Man... What is a man?

A man takes care of his responsibilities, not afraid to stand up to anything that'll compromise his home stability. Tryna build a legacy that last forever...like Jesus against the Pharisees. A man doesn't need validation, only clarification on the promise given to him from the one in charge of his creation. A man can have emotions, that he's not afraid to show, he puts others before himself. But there's something else you should know...REAL MEN DO CRY! Due to a lot of different subjects I couldn't fit in this sentence. Now ladies, I'd like to come to you in a form of repentance: I'm sorry for all the men that ever hurt you, abused your virtue, that you lost yourself to, that made you give up on guys, give up on love, give up on God. I'm sorry for all the whack dudes with the "nice guy facades." Just know you're beautiful, and that's from God, not me but it takes a real man to have the vision to see. Peace.

• • • • • •

**I polled my community asking what they thought makes a man, and this was their response:**

- Takes on another kid not their own, sticks up for what's right, a gentleman (chivalry), a Man of God
- Maturity, gets things done, emotions don't cloud judgment
- Compassion, open/vulnerability, leader (no crack), strong beliefs
- Responsible, strength of character, boldness, assertiveness
- Responsible, provider, owns up to wrongs, considers himself a man
- Mental fortitude
- Chivalry, paying for dates, masculinity, taking charge, God-fearing, honesty, breadwinner
- Honest, loyal, no excuses, responsible, selfless, courageous
- Responsible
- Integrity
- A man to me is a male that takes care of responsibility and has his own, mature mindset

• • • • • •

# GRACELAND

Lord I love you, and your love's deeper than the ocean. It goes past the point of emotions. It drowns out the world's commotion when I'm distracted and only focused on my own life's constant motion. I don't care what people think. Yes, they're gonna judge me surely, but it's whatever, I just want your holy name to get the glory. The only reason I'm sharing my heart with you is cuz I know somebody needs to hear my story. And if I shed a couple tears, I don't want you to feel sorry. See, these tears are me just overwhelmed by the love that he has for me. This ain't about no damn religion, but yes, I'm Christian and I ain't perfect, but my dad still shows me love and keeps me even when I don't deserve it. I drink, smoke, have sex and God still says I'm worth it. When I turned my back on him, he still blessed me with purpose. I learned I'm not my sins or my mistakes, cuz he greets his child with patience. And cuz I have a dad like him there is no condemnation, so I can turn from sin and lay eyes on him and embrace the grace he placed in my life and I can keep on running this race called life I'm racing, Amen.

# WHERE DO I START?

## Part 1

I want to share with you something that's really on my heart, but when I try to write this thing I ain't know where to start.

We were holding on to each other and that was my first thought.

Me losing you to forever that was my second thought.

The word forever led me right back to my first thought, love how you used to gas me up but now my car is parked. And in my life learned lessons, love is something I wasn't taught. You kissed me, then said let's be friends. Now what should be my thoughts?

Trying to be cool with you on this oh let's be friends trip but I can't stop thinking about our intimate relationship. I don't know why I just can't seem to see me over it.

Explosiveness left me emotionless and now I'm motion sick on roller coasters that I'm rolling with. If my heart had controllers, you're controlling it: up, down and around and around, and when you touch me you slow motion it.

We juvenile and I'm a delinquent. How I'm approaching it. If you back that thang up Imma show you just what the potion is, but now you over it. Didn't realize that I was blowing it. If I did something wrong you wasn't showing it. Wish you'd just tell me what the problem is.

Whatever it takes to right the wrongs I didn't know about. They call those mistakes.

# Part 2

Trying to find the words don't know where to start

Picking up the pieces of my broken heart.

Tell me what to do to be the man for you. If you write me the plan girl I swear I'll see it through.

I just got in a lyft to come give me your mind body spirit and soul a lift and get it equipped with a love you once thought you were unfit for.

As your dad walked out the door and your ex walked in, left your heart in a whirlwind and caused you to break your back when it was only supposed to bend. Now you can't accept the love I'm trying to give you cuz of the condition your heart's been left in.

But I'm willing to take the chance, roll the dice, shoot my shot blindfolded with one arm tied behind my back because you're worth it.

And if I spread the moments of my life out on the timeline of eternity, the moment that I met you would be in the center of it all. And if I could run right back to it I would, but your love is so strong it makes me weak so I'd probably have to crawl in when I get there. I'll hold on to your heart so tight that even if you slip I'll never let you fall.

• • • • • •

# I CAN'T WAIT

Met her at the job,

back when I used to rob,

not money or jewelry but the hearts I used to throb.

I'm sure you heard about the sobs,

some chicks say I'm a fraud

but using tricks to poke and prod didn't work out on this type
of broad.

The shoulders is what she went for. I followed her out of the
door. My approach was rather simple.

Can I get yo name and number and we can speak a lil bit more.

She said my name is J but the number you have to work for.

Cool, so how bout you tell me about yourself. She said, do you
want to know or are you looking to get felt……. on?

Her response was the quiet before the storm.

Should've listened but in my head, I was sure that my game was
strong.

So, the game continues on.

She said, let me ask you something, if you was my man, and that
was the plan, then tell me what morals you standin' on. Let
me know that before this thing lingers on.

And from that night I know she changed my life. I was looking
to dog her out, now I'm thinkin' that she's my wife.

# BURN ONE (THE ONE)

I wish that you could see your own smile, cuz when I see it, I
    grin
heart breaks in two if I see you frown.
Just let me know what happened.
I know one thing and that is for sure,
since you've been mine my life seems worth so much more
And I used to cry every night, until I looked in your eyes.
(You're my wildest dream come true).
I am the luckiest man alive.
My world was stuck now it spins.
You showed and taught me who I was,
with your love.
I'd give you my heart, I'd jump off a cliff,
if it meant you could live.
You're so (Beautiful) you sit inside Heaven's gaze,
and then I smell your fragrance and it drives me insane.
Your love is like the perfect stain.
Even through all of the pain,
I'm forever loving you!

• • • • • •

# NOTHING IN MIND

I decided to write this with nothing in mind, similar to your thoughts concerning me, nothing. And I made sure every line in this one didn't run on. And there's a reason for that period: I wanted to prove that I was enough, to me. As I sit here listening to control, I can't stop thinking about how my emotions are constantly under yours. And then you walked past, the inspiration for this entry. You didn't speak or notice or even see me, but do you ever? I don't know. You ever hear the saying, "The person you want doesn't want you, but the people you don't want do"? I have a hard time believing that because when I think about it, I never really wanted you. I wanted you to have the thought of me so I can have the option of being important to you, then I choose not to be because I've always been too afraid to show you me.

● ● ● ● ● ●

# SORRY

I'm sorry for being selfish,

I'm sorry for not loving you,

I'm sorry for hurting you,

I'm sorry for not treating you like the queen you are.

All I know how to be is sorry.

I clearly can't be the man you want or need or deserve, so I guess I'll just be SORRY.

# KILL ~ STEAL ~ DESTROY

Day one: Another one born, small, fragile and has a beautiful smile. I thought he was average, but I can't put him in that file. God thinks he's special and he loves him, well that ain't my style. I'll get him while he's young, so first his self-esteem I'll defile. I'll start with what he sees. I'll put unrealistic images and glamorized lifestyles on his TVs. He'll start to think that's what he has to be. He'll give his very last breath to try and live out those fantasies. Oh! And while I'm at it, let's bring in some big guns, because I can't let you know who wins. How about this? I'll introduce him to the lustful sin. Lust will go a long way with this one. Well hey, doesn't it with everyone? It did with his dad, so why don't we keep it all in the family, shall we? This kid loves games, so with that I'll cunningly put sex in the frame. As his dad leaves him in the car all alone, with his cell phone, he'll go to play games on it. As time passes his attention span can't take it. His curiosity will lead him right to the pit. As he scrolls through the phone what does he find? In the video section a woman moaning, with a man right behind. He hurries and backs out, not sure what he just saw. Doesn't matter: it's in his subconscious. I'll use that for his fall. Over and over, little by little, I condition his mind, shape his thoughts, dictate his actions. Yeah, this one is mine. He wonders and ponders until his mind takes him to another one of many tools, the internet. He looks up what he knows nothing about. He has questions, and I'll help him get all the answers he wants. I'll educate him on this thing called sex, in the most pressing and aggressive way I know how. I'll teach him women are just objects for his enjoyment, and that sex is meaningless. That way, as he finds many different partners, he'll unknowingly be splitting himself into several broken pieces. God can't use what's not whole, right? Right! He's thirteen now, so I'll finally get to expose him first-hand. I'll sink this boy faster than an elephant in quicksand. Get him an older girl. I also have under my thumb, to lend him a hand, and her lips and her tongue, oh this will be fun. He finally did it, yes. The deed has been done, but this lifelong vice has just begun.

# CHAPTER FIVE
# SERMONS/REVELATIONS

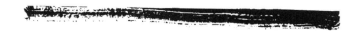

I've included this part in the book to show the role God has played in my life and how spending mass amounts of time with him has shaped me to be the man I am today. Here you will find notes and spiritual downloads I've received from God regarding potential sermons. Some were for a Bible study group I led a few times at AMDA, and the others are essentially real and transparent conversations/dialog with God. I believe this section may help you be more transparent in your communication with God and yourself.

• • • • • •

# My Encounter with God (6/15/2017)

He told me to lay down on my couch with a blanket on. After laying in silence for about 10 minutes, I felt his presence surround me and my spirit and physical body were temporarily semi disconnected. He began to move my hand as my eyes were closed. He showed me his hand grabbing mine and guiding it across my torso. I then became scared and opened my eyes. I then told him to have his way and I trusted him. I closed my eyes again and this time I kept hearing in my mind my spirit speaking in tongues. Slowly my physical body began speaking very quietly. I then felt as if I were floating. I asked why he was moving my hand before me, and he said, "Because I want you to go write something down."

I said, "What?"

He answered me, "I will write, you just go."

I continued to lay there, and he then raised his voice three times, saying "Go!" After that he said, "Why are you not moving?"

I then got up and went to the table where my journal and pen were. He took over from there. Through me he picked up the pen and opened the journal. I closed my eyes and the first thing he told me to write was the letter D. Soon after he put two words in my head: disciple and discipline. He then began to freely move the pen about, and he drew constant infinity symbols. He then took the pen and went down across to the left up into a loop back up right across then back up. He drew an arm that represented my arm. I then opened my eyes to see what he made. It wasn't until just now as I write this that he told me what it all means. The D is next to the infinity symbols, meaning his disciples (believers) will live forever in eternity, but we must always practice discipline while on earth. The infinity symbols go into the arm picture and they are where a hand would be on the end of an arm. This means the works of my hand in line with God's purpose will last forever.

After the drawing he told me he is my Father, I am his son and I am great for that reason alone. He then placed a robe on me to say I was a king. I felt it, so I began to open my eyes. He immediately said, "Close your eyes. This is not about what you can see in the physical, but what you can see in the spirit."

After that he took my left hand and slid it across the Bible. He said, "This is my body." I began to speak in tongues again for a time after that. We talked a bit more, and he then said, "I am finished," and I returned to my normal state of being.

· · · · · ·

# Who I am? (12/23/2017)

- God, speak to me more clearly regarding my relationship with my girlfriend. What should we be focusing on together, and what are we pursuing in this present time and within the next year?

- God, please guide and prepare me as your vessel to be used in these upcoming Bible studies. I ask that you constantly humble me so that it is your words that come off my lips and they fall onto soft hearts with love.

- Thank you God for connecting me to more and more of your people every day. I see clearly that you are using me as a focal point to connect all the believers here in this immediate community, so continue to renew my spiritual eyes and discernment to be led by you and effectively be of service to your people.

- Lord, I ask that you make clear what the purpose of my relationships are. I know you allow me to connect to certain people for a reason, and I believe that certain people are purpose-made, so Lord, reveal that purpose, thank you. Amen.

- Lord, bless me with an abundance of opportunities to talk to you and about you and your love. Continue to use me and my life more than ever before, and to be an example of what life with you is, and what pure love is in the community and world.

- If I'm being honest God, I've been putting this off, and I'm a little nervous to outright ask you who I am, because I am afraid of what you are going to tell me. It may not be something that I want to hear, but I come boldly to you and I am ready for you to tell me exactly who I am to you, and who I am to this world in regards to the work that you would have me do.

## I AM
- Pastor
- Prophet
- Husband
- Righteousness of God
- Dancer
- Actor
- Minister
- Worshipper
- Healer
- Some people are not going to hear about the truth of Jesus unless I tell them
- Refuge
- Choreographer
- Prayer Warrior
- I am about to be up against spiritual opposition, and I will WIN over a sorcerer. (Glory to God for knowing what I

can handle with his spirit that enables me)
- Prophetic Vessel
- Demon Killer

Thank you, Heavenly Father, for being here with me and speaking to me. Continue to make known to me the mysteries of your vastness and the plans for my life. Continue to develop into something the love and purposeful relationship between me and others that you have placed in my life. Give us daily instructions and objectives that will achieve the glory of your Kingdom. Let us not be torn away or be led astray by temptation or distraction, but let us be moved, filled and led by your spirit and that alone. I thank you for the victory in this upcoming season of spiritual warfare. I decree and declare the enemy has no foothold or space in my life nor my atmosphere, and he will flee at the sound of my voice. Even as I write this prayer, he is trembling like the punk that he is. Thank you for the boldness and fire you planted in me Jesus, and until the day I die and even beyond then, I will worship, honor and glorify your name. Make my path narrow and straight, and speak clearly to me Lord in all situations I go through in my life. Jesus, Holy Spirit, lead me and guide me. Be the center of my life, forever in Jesus' mighty name I pray. Hallelujah, amen, amen and amen!

● ● ● ● ● ●

# Conversation with GOD (12/14/2017)

I am currently in a season of being built up. God, I feel you constantly speaking and revealing wisdom and spiritual knowledge to me just as I asked. Thank you for that. In terms of my relationship with my girlfriend, we've made our mistakes and now I feel we're being torn apart because of it. God, heal my unbelief and the doubt that comes when we have arguments. I know that she is for me. Remove the part of me that has the unreal expectation of "perfect" in this relationship. Show me how not to let our emotions tear us apart, and make your loving spirit draw us closer. I rebuke any plans the enemy has to cause division among us and lay hold of the divine joint plan you have for the both of us. Thank you, Jesus.

• • • • • •

# Know Thy Patterns (2/17/2018)

- Whenever I feel lonely, I look for a female that I'm attracted to, to be around.
- I usually feel lonely at night between 8:00 PM and 2:00 AM.
- Every girl I pursue is outside of the body of Christ and views me as a "nice guy."
- I often try to uphold an image of having it all together.
- When I want attention, I go to school and flirt with girls who I know will play into it.

- When I can't get company, I usually just watch Netflix.
- When I hear of parties I wasn't invited to, I begin to feel as if nobody likes me and no one cares about me or cares to be around me. I also feel like people don't see my value.
- The more hurt I feel in my relationship, the easier it is for me to push away from God. I have equated my spiritual growth to my relationship with my girlfriend.

● ● ● ● ● ●

## Why Do I Feel Rejection from Peers Socially?

In elementary school I formed a very-tight knit group who were the most popular kids at school. There was me and three other guys and we all had girlfriends, and at the time we were the IT crowd. We were so close that we pretty much did everything together: recess, lunch, fieldtrips, sitting in class – all of us were always together. In fourth grade I believe is when things changed. Up to that point, I had a very big ego and a false sense of importance. I was smart, popular, I had a girlfriend, and everyone seemed to like me. All of that started to change when my best friend had to move to Delaware. We wound up losing a member of our group. Soon after, the summer going into fifth grade, my girlfriend was moving to another place as well. And back then social media did not exist so the only social interaction we had was at school, meaning if you weren't at the same school then that person pretty much didn't exist. So, at this point in my life is when it kind of turned to shambles. Not only had two members of my clique left, but the couples were starting to break up and switching, so it was confusing and chaotic for us all. To make things worse, after some time of being in a long-distance relationship, my girlfriend wound up breaking up with me, and then a day or two later I found out that she had been talking to my best friend over the phone and they seemed to have become a thing. I felt like it was the ultimate betrayal. It was my first heartbreak. Looking back, I can say that all those events were the root of my being scared of being rejected, because the friends I held so dearly and who I thought would last forever were stripped from me, and that bruised and cracked my inner mirror for sure, especially as it relates to friendships and relationships in general.

* * * * * *

## Silent but Godly (Living While God Has You Hidden)

March 25th, 2017 was the date that I truly dedicated my soul and my life to Jesus and God, but it wasn't the first time I'd been saved or baptized. I grew up in the Church and felt God's call very early on my life. I have been saved since I was about seven or eight years old. I knew Jesus was truth and I accepted him as my savior, but for most of my adolescent life I tried doing life my way. I was a good kid on paper: decent grades, well behaved, respectful, well spoken, everything that a young kid should be, right? However, outside the scope of parents, adults and authority figures, I got into a whole lot of what, for lack of a better word, I call "stuff." I was introduced to sex and drugs very early, at about 13 years old. At age 13 I got involved with two females who I eventually allowed to take me down a dark path.

• • • • • • •

## Lust (Living Under Satan's Temptations)

This specific section looks at lust as a whole and all that comes with it. This is not a bashing of homosexual people, but an unveiling of truth. Sin has no scale: one sin is never greater or less than another. And sin is put as simply as missing the mark in regard to the standard of living that God desires and requires of us in Him.

> *"For I wrote you out of great distress and anguish of heart and with many tears, not to grieve you but to let you know the depth of my love for you."*
> ***2 Corinthians 2:4, NIV***

> *"So I tell you this, and insist on it in the LORD, that you must no longer live as the Gentiles do, in the futility of their thinking. [18]They are darkened in their understanding and separated from the life of God because of the ignorance that is in them due to the hardening of their hearts. [19]Having lost all sensitivity, they have given themselves over to sensuality so as to indulge in every kind of impurity, and they are full of greed."*
> ***Ephesians 4:17-19, NIV***

- We must step out of our old ways of thinking first to start change. You can't just fall into ungodly activities just because everyone else is. That means your circle of friends might need to change.
- The more you ignore the spirit man you have telling you things are wrong, the easier it is to do wrong and not feel wrong. Stop muting your spirit man.
- Ignorance equals lack of knowledge.
- Futility equals pointless, emptiness, fruitlessness.

> *"You were taught, with regard to your former way of life,*
> *to put off your old self, which is being corrupted by its*
> *deceitful desires."*
> **Ephesians 4:22, NIV**

There is no good in the old life you had before Christ. You were living solely off the desires of your flesh, which is completely insatiable.

> *"Do not let any unwholesome talk come out of your*
> *mouths, but only what is helpful for building others up according to their needs, that it may benefit those who listen."*
> **Ephesians 4:29, NIV**

> *"Not only so, but we also glory in our sufferings, because*
> *we know that suffering produces perseverance;*
> *perseverance, character; and character, hope."*
> **Romans 5:3-4, NIV**

- You must no longer engage in sex talks or hook up stories or any of that. Be courageous to either shut the convo down or remove yourself. Make it known to others that you are no longer willing to be a part of convos like those.
- That type of talk opens your spirit to the spirit of lust, and it will sit there in your mind and you'll start to think about sex and get all heated up.
- The Holy Spirit and God are not of those or in those conversations.
- Ephesians 6:12 – We must understand that the lust and urges we feel are all fleshly and there are spirits attached to them.
- Spirits can linger in certain places where sexual immorality has taken place from convos, to actual acts or people.
- We must, through the power of God in Jesus, rebuke and remove them out of our space that we occupy.

• • • • • •

## Homosexuality

- Generational curses
- Pushed to it through broken relationships i.e., significant others or parents

*"The wrath of God is being revealed from Heaven against all the godlessness and wickedness of people, who suppress the truth by their wickedness, since what may be known*

*about God is plain to them, because God has made it plain to them. For since the creation of the world God's invisible qualities-his eternal power and divine nature-have been clearly seen, being understood from what has been made, so that people are without excuse. For although they knew God, they neither glorified him as God nor gave thanks to him, but their thinking became futile and their foolish hearts were darkened. Although they claimed to be wise, they became fools and exchanged the glory of the immortal God for images made to look like a mortal human being and birds and animals and reptiles. Therefore God gave them over in the sinful desires of their hearts to sexual impurity for the degrading of their bodies with one another. They exchanged the truth about God for a lie and worshiped and served created things rather than the Creator-who is forever praised. Amen. Because of this, God gave them over to shameful lusts. Even their women exchanged natural sexual relations for unnatural ones."*
**Romans 1:18-26, NIV**

• • • • • •

## The Enemy Was Pulling Them Away from All God Promised to Them (Abraham)

Romans 1:18-19 – God is opposed to all forms of wickedness and is beginning to impose wrath. He's upset because they turn away from God even though he has shown himself and his goodness.

**Romans 1:21** – The people refuse to glorify God and are committed to a foolish lifestyle, worshipping everything but God.

**Romans 1:24-26** – God then gave the people over to their sin and their desire for sexual impurity in which they begin degrading each other. He allowed the people to be overtaken by shameful lust. Women lusted after women and men after men.

> *"Although they know God's righteous decree that those who do such things deserve death, they not only continue to do these very things but also approve of those who practice them."*
> ***Romans 1:32, NIV***

Although the people knew God's righteousness they continued to turn away and instead they approved and glorified those who practice wrongdoing and sexual immorality.

> *"Do not offer any part of yourself to sin as an instrument of wickedness, but rather offer yourselves to God as those who have been brought from death to life; and offer every part of yourself to him as an instrument of righteousness. ¹⁴For sin shall no longer be your master, because you are not under the law, but under grace. ¹⁵What then? Shall we sin because we are not under the law but under grace?*

> *By no means! ¹⁶Don't you know that when you offer yourselves to someone as obedient slaves, you are slaves of the one you obey-whether you are slaves to sin, which leads to death, or to obedience, which leads to righteousness? ¹⁷But thanks be to God that, though you used to be slaves to sin, you have come to obey from your heart the pattern of teaching that has now claimed your allegiance. ¹⁸You have been set free from sin and have become slaves to righteousness."*
> ***Romans 6:13-18, NIV***

**Belt of truth**: Knowing God's truth is the way we deny and conquer over Satan's lies and deception.

**Breastplate of righteousness**: To constantly repent for sins and do what is right in the eyes of God. Meditate on his law.

**Feet fitted with gospel of peace**: Be eager to preach and share the gospel and good news of God.

**Shield of faith**: Faith protects us because we believe our God covers us even when we don't see it. Absolute conviction that he will do what he promised.

> *"Now faith is confidence in what we hope for and assurance about what we do not see."*
> ***Hebrews 11:1, NIV***

**Helmet of Salvation**: Remember and focus on the incredible sacrifice of Jesus and its importance and goal to save us and our souls. Protects our mind from discouragement and despair.

**Sword of the spirit**: This is the living word of God. The word of God applies in any situation. Its knowledge gives us authority and power, for it is written. Standing firm in the word of God defeats Satan easily. One must study consistently.

> Now the serpent was more crafty than any of the wild animals the LORD God had made. He said to the woman, "Did God really say, 'You must not eat from any tree in the garden'?"
>
> The woman said to the serpent, "We may eat fruit from the trees in the garden, but God did say, 'You must not eat fruit from the tree that is in the middle of the garden, and you must not touch it, or you will die.'"
>
> "You will not certainly die," the serpent said to the woman. "For God knows that when you eat from it your eyes will be opened, and you will be like God, knowing good and evil."
>
> When the woman saw that the fruit of the tree was good for food and pleasing to the eye, and also desirable for gaining wisdom, she took some and ate it. She also gave some to her husband, who was with her, and he ate it.

*Then the eyes of both of them were opened, and they realized they were naked; so they sewed fig leaves together and made coverings for themselves.*

*Then the man and his wife heard the sound of the LORD God as he was walking in the garden in the cool of the day, and they hid from the LORD God among the trees of the garden. But the LORD God called to the man, "Where are you?"*

*He answered, "I heard you in the garden, and I was afraid because I was naked; so I hid."*

*And he said, "Who told you that you were naked? Have you eaten from the tree that I commanded you not to eat from?"*

*The man said, "The woman you put here with me – she gave me some fruit from the tree, and I ate it."*

**Genesis 3: 1-12, NIV**

● ● ● ● ● ●

## You Know You Wrong

1. **Why Are You Entertaining the Enemy?**
   A. Oftentimes we allow the enemy to speak, and we listen instead of immediately rebuking him and silencing his voice, which is full of deception.

B. One must be able to discern the voice of God, our own voice, and words from Satan.

2. **You must not eat, you must not touch, or you will die**
   A. We often try to walk a tightrope with the will of God. We try to tiptoe and beat God on technicalities. We will dabble in stuff and say, "Oh I touched it, but I didn't eat it," trying to justify.

   Me and my girlfriend knew we couldn't have sex, but in our lust we'd give each other oral sex and say, "Oh but that's not really sex, we didn't have intercourse."

3. **Fix Your Eyesight**
   A. When the woman saw that the fruit was good for food and pleasing to the eye, everything she made her decision off in regard to eating the fruit was fleshly appeal.
   B. We must operate in a way that puts our spirit first, before our flesh. When we look at things, ask God, "Please reveal if this is what I want or what you want God. I know this feels good, but am I hurting you while I do this? Is this pushing me toward life and righteousness or to self-indulgence and death?

   For a long time, I had a problem of the lust of the eyes. I just could not turn away from looking at female's bodies. I'd look and then sometimes stare or fantasize over their breasts or bottom, and those thoughts became manifest into lustful dreams. I would be so confused, asking my-self why I was having those dreams, trying to blame the enemy when really it was me. It wasn't until I got honest with myself and God that I was able to check myself and be free from this.

## 4. Take Responsibility for What You Have Done

A. God said, "Have you eaten from the tree that I com-manded you not to eat from?" The man said, "The woman you put here with me – she gave me some fruit from the tree, and I ate it."

Don't throw blame on other people. As humans, we hate being wrong. We hate getting caught doing some-thing we know we shouldn't be doing. Remember as a kid when you got in trouble in school, and you'd be in awe because the other kid you were throwing stuff with didn't and the teacher says I didn't see them I saw you. I believe God is that same way. When dealing with you he isn't concerned with what other people did, he wants to correct and fix you. He chases those he loves.

● ● ● ● ● ●

# What is Prayer?

• Legal authority and Dominion of earth given to humans (Genesis 1:27).

- Prayer gives permission for divine / spiritual intervention from God, into earthly matters.
- The word was with God, and the word was God (John 1).
- Prayer is conversation with God, not a monologue.

# CHAPTER SIX
# CONTRARY TO POPULAR BELIEF

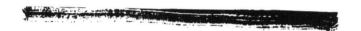

**Part 1**

To be completely honest, this has been the hardest thing I have ever written about. I have no problem speaking of my wild, crazy, teenage high school adventures: from sneaking out of my best friend's house at three in the morning and essentially stealing his mom's car to go to parties in the city; to me smoking weed at an excess of at least five blunts a day; and even my not so brief period of depression and suicidal thoughts that crept into my mind all throughout middle school and into high school. But what I am about to write now is harder than all the aforementioned. It's hard because for most of my life after it, I blocked it out. It's hard because I knew it wasn't me or who God created me to be, but the guilt I felt from it walked and held my hand every day. It's hard because I'm sometimes afraid that, if I tell this part of my truth and my story, a lot of people will distance themselves from me. Relationships will be tainted with this hazed view of who I am, and that some people who so aggressively tried to ruin my social reputation will feel some sick sense of satisfaction to know they were "right" about it all. The only way I'm able to write it now is because I know I am not my actions, and I am only who and what God says I am. I have been blessed to grow from my experiences, and I believe that me sharing this story will be the life vest to many people who feel like they are drowning in the waters of their shameful secrets.

This is about my adolescent experiments with homosexuality. This is often seen as taboo, especially as a black boy who played all the sports, who talked to all the girls, whose dad and brother outwardly made it apparent that being gay was the worst thing in the world, and as a CHRISTIAN. From the time I was about 15 or 16 years old (eighth grade) until my second semester of college, I often went back and forth with the idea that I might be gay. Although I never had a very intimate relationship with a guy, I did some things that made me question myself on more than one occasion.

Between the ages of 15 and 19 I had sexual experiences with four boys. Three of them I received oral sex from, and the fourth I spent extended periods of time with in which we kissed and just hung out. Now I know this information is a huge shock for some. It is also an "I told you so" for others. I've already shared this with a couple of people who I trust the most, and it will come as no surprise to them. As I continue to go in depth on these experiences, how they made me feel and what I learned from each of them, I want to remind you all that this is to help those who are currently or have been in this stage of their life and are scared. Understand that everything that God has "allowed" you to go through can and will be used for your good, and no matter what you do, you will never be outside or too far from God's love for you, regardless of what people say. I quoted the word "allowed" because I want to be clear that God will never DO anything negative or harmful to you, nor will he ever wish for you to go through these things. However, in our ignorance as humans who are prone to mistakes and sin due to ignorance and the world in which we were born into we all go through. God allows us to experience these things in the hopes that we will come to him and accept him as our Father who gives unconditional love and guidance to his children.

From this point on I will no longer try to justify my actions or try to save face. I am writing all fact, and from genuine experience regardless of fear of judgment, whether that be from, family, friends, or strangers. God needs me to speak this truth and so I will.

I believe the first time someone ever called me gay was maybe in about eighth grade. As kids we were fed this toxic homophobic juice that we sipped at every meal, breakfast, lunch and dinner. I was put into a dance class that was a mandatory art credit my eighth-grade year of middle school. Of course, as one of the boys in the class, I was automatically being called gay by all the other boys in school. Now at the time I really didn't even know what being gay meant, but I knew it was something that was unacceptable, and I had to immediately defend myself at all cost to not be associated with that word.

My first homosexual encounter happened with a boy named Dominic as I transitioned out of middle school. Dominic was a year older than me and he went to a different school, but we lived in the same neighborhood. Dominic first reached out to me on the social media website, MySpace. Eventually he and I started to hang out around our neighborhood. He was openly gay but not extremely flamboyant, so I figured there was no harm in kicking it with him. One day Dominic expressed his attraction to me. Although I was not attracted to him, that feeling of being wanted was like a drug that I had never really tasted. Prior to him, I had had relationships with females before. I lost my virginity around 14 years old, about seventh grade, but nobody ever really wanted me the way he wanted me. As I look back on it now, lust was a very big factor in the entirety of our relationship, but at the time I had no knowledge of what lust was and the effects it had on me.

One day, Dominic and I were hanging around his apartment building complex when we decided that we were going to smoke weed using a pipe he had bought at the mall a few days prior. We smoked, and then he asked if I wanted to come over to his place, which was right there. I said yes, and so we went. I will say, that as I recall, I had full knowledge of what was going on and what could potentially happen. We went into his room, and I sat on his bed and he sat on the floor. We started to watch TV, and then he put his back up against the bed and I started to mess with him, pushing and hitting him. I then asked him if he ever had sex with a girl, and he told me yes, but that he liked sex with guys better. He then said that it's better with guys, and then he asked if he could give me oral. I hesitated for a second. I remember justifying to myself that oral sex is still oral sex no matter who is giving it to you, and that it didn't matter that he was a boy, I just wanted to be pleasured. I agreed to his request, and that is what happened. Afterward, I went home feeling this undeniable and unexplainable shame and regret that I had not ever felt before and knowing that I could never tell anyone what had happened.

A few weeks later I began to hear the rumors circulating around that I was gay and that I had sex with a boy. Of course I fought extremely hard to renounce such accusations although I knew them to be true. I was genuinely scared of what others would say and think of me. I was also very worried because I knew that I liked girls and wanted to have girlfriends, but I was sure that if everyone knew the truth about this situation then the whole girlfriend thing was out the window with no bungee cord. My reputation, the fear of judgment all weighed on me so heavily that I completely cut Dominic off and I still up to this day have never seen or spoken to him.

• • • • • •

## Part 2

This is about the last time I did or experienced anything sexual with another guy. My first year of college had begun and I was still the young, immature, and lust-driven kid I was in high school. I must make it so clear how powerful lust is. I'd even suggest that it is right up there with fear. It has the incredible ability to make people do things that may seem irrational or even out of character. Combine that with the influence of any drug or substance and there is no telling the outcome. I wanted to say that so that people reading this can really take a step back and analyze where in their lives they may have let lust control their actions and/or decisions.

I know since I was about 13, lust has impacted my decision making constantly and consistently. Throughout most of my adolescence I made a ton of choices that were determined entirely by the desire to get into a position to have sex with people. It got to a point that I had developed a system. I had it down pat. From about the end of my tenth-grade year in high school until about my second year of college, I was an absolute mess. I had sex with many people in many different situations. Lust had become the undeniable driving motivation for almost all the actions I took. Naturally having the gift of speaking, wit, persuasion and being able to tell what people wanted or desired, I was an avid manipulator who could talk my way into just about any sexual situation that I wanted with just about anyone I pleased. I operated on this set of rules and standards until it finally caught up with me and all came to a head.

By the time I was in my second semester of college I had developed an intimate relationship with a woman who'd eventually become my girlfriend. The relationship started with me pursuing her just as I did with any other female, but soon and totally unexpectedly, I fell in love with this girl. Now the fact that I fell in love with her did not automatically cancel out my issue of lust. I think it is important to say that, because a lot of us often think, *Oh if I could just get this thing or get with the RIGHT ONE, then I'd stop messing around or like you've heard, "being a hoe."* Just because you found something good does not mean that your other problems will simply disappear, and that goes with everything – relationships, money, everything. It's like someone who is bad with managing their finances. They'd say if they had a million dollars it would solve all their problems. In actuality, they'd probably blow it on all the same things they always blew money on, just on a larger scale, and without a doubt would go right back to being broke again.

That was me in this new relationship. I loved this woman, but I still lusted over other females, and even allowed my lust to drive me to having another sexual relationship with a guy. So, this was at the beginning of our relationship. We weren't boyfriend and girlfriend, but we were supposed to be exclusive. I clearly allowed my lust to let me not honor that at all. There was a guy who, just as happened years before with Dominic, made clear his interest in me. I still loved the feeling of being wanted and desired, so of course I fed into it and all the sexual jokes and light-hearted flirtation we did that stayed just between us.

One weekend he asked if I wanted to come to his house and spend the weekend there. I agreed and we went. Now I also think it's important for us to recognize the patterns and cycles of our dysfunctions and vices/sins. The enemy has no new tricks, all he does is tap into the holes we have in our lives based on the sin we were born into or opened ourselves up to, and the trauma or generational curses that have manifested in our lives. He sets up cycle after cycle after cycle to keep us trapped and living in our sin, so much that we don't even realize it and we get to a point where we just say, "Oh it's normal, it's always been that way," not understanding that we don't have to live below who we really were called to be by accepting a sub-standard way of living. So I went over to this guy's house and, long story short, one night I let him give me oral sex. It was again still shameful for me and something that I had vowed to never share with anyone.

Some weeks later, the woman who I was involved with was now my girlfriend. Her having such incredible discernment and wisdom, she asked if I ever had sex with guys. I wanted to be honest, but I was scared to tell her that I did when I was already with her, so I only confessed to the times that had happened years before when I was in high school.

Sometime later, after I had been home for a break, when I returned to school, I was greeted with some news I did not want to hear. Rumors started to circulate that I had sex with the guy. Of course my girlfriend immediately defended me, but she wasn't naïve. We wound up going to her place and she straight up asked me what was up. I broke down in tears and finally told her the truth of the situation. I cried for two reasons. The first was that I was exposed. I was terrified of how people would now view me, but more than that I was truly scared of being vulnerable like that. For a long time, the lies and half-truths I lived behind in my mind kept me safe, comfortable and away from a cruel world. The second reason I cried was due to the fact that I knew how much I had absolutely crushed the woman that I was in love with. I knew all the thoughts running in her head. Was the guy she loved gay? I knew the harshness of the words she would hear from others, people saying how dumb she was and so on. I felt terrible for that and what I put her through.

She then had a choice to make. She could choose to just flat out leave me and cut me out her life or stay. Her being one of the strongest, amazing, most God-fearing women I know, she decided to put her feelings aside and show me love the way God loves me. She saw through the lens of God and looked past my actions and decided to see my real issue, to see the scared, insecure, lust-driven little boy I was, and she allowed God to use her for my healing.

This moment, in combination with a few others, was one of the driving factors that led me back to Christ and living my life for

Him again after doing my own thing for so, so long. Without her allowing God to use her as a vessel the way he did, I know my life wouldn't be what it is now, and I'd have gone through even more heartache than what I have.

I needed to write these two stories for a couple reasons. I had to share my story and my truth so that other people would be able to push past fear and shame to recognize their truth. I want people, and more importantly men, to understand that no matter what we've done or gone through, including but not limited to homosexuality or "gay things," that you are not what you may have done no matter what outside people say. I want people to see the very thing that you thought disqualified you, is the very thing that God uses to qualify you. No matter what your family or friends or anyone else may say, I know it's hard to block out the negativity, but it is possible, by tapping into the unlimited love that God has for you.

Now I must address the people with the toxically engrained mental position of homophobia. Contrary to popular belief, it is possible for anyone, but more specifically a man, to have sexual experiences with the same sex and still be "straight." I am an example of that, and I am absolutely no longer ashamed of what I have done because I know God uses everything for my good in the end. I used to look at what I did as this immeasurable weight of shame and guilt for the things I did with guys, but now I see those things as a blessing. I view it as a blessing because of his GRACE. I may have not been able to experience God's love the way I did. It is also a blessing, because I now have another way and tool to use in my pursuit of bringing all glory to God. I am and will continue to be used in whatever way God wants, especially my weaknesses. I am proud to be the one God uses to speak on topics such as these. I feel honored he chose me and that he gives me strength I don't have, DAILY, to carry out the purpose he set for me.

I also want to speak to the people who may read this and think I am a homophobic Christian who is against all gay people. That is the absolute furthest from the truth. I love everybody because God loves me despite all the messed-up things I've done. I believe that we are all of God's creation and we are not what we do or our sexual preference. There is nothing that we could ever possibly do that will separate us from His love. Sex is sex and sin is sin, no matter the gender. A man and a woman having sex outside of marriage is just as bad as two people of the same sex. Please don't be fooled into thinking it is not. Sin doesn't come with a weight attached. You can't only get a little bit of sin like you weigh produce at the grocery store. It is what it is. I hate the sin, but I LOVE the sinner. I am a sinner and God still uses me and loves me just as he does anybody willing to receive. Jesus' blood covers us from the punishment of sin so that we would have the opportunity to come to him and God and live as we were created, to be our best self, to live abundantly and experience true, genuine, unmerited LOVE. Each day we have a choice to be better or worse than the day before, I hope these stories and the rest of this book inspire you to be better and live a life worth living, and one that has eternal and generational impact for the better.

# CHAPTER SEVEN
# UNABRIDGED

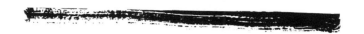

These are some of my day to day thoughts and feelings while navigating my first years of college, expressed raw and unedited.

• • • • • •

## 1/12/17

**Really Good Moments** – Today is a Thursday and has had some really good moments. I recently, since I came back from break, have had this "kill shit" mentality. All week I haven't been overthinking in my dance classes.

I have been "just dancing" and not only am I feeling great about the work I'm doing, but my teachers say I'm doing really well too. Last night I auditioned a duet piece for Raise the Barre. Unfortunately, I didn't get selected, but I am totally okay with that. We didn't execute how we should have, but again it's okay and I'm learning that every "no" is an extra push. Ru (my girl-friend) told me that God isn't going to put me out until I'm ready and the moment is right, so until then I'll continue to work and create and grow.

I did well in ballet, but the highlight of my day was my DTP class with Nicole Berger. It's part of the reason I'm so okay with not being chosen for RTB. Nicole's piece is so refreshing, and it feels so light and effortless and reminds me "I can dance." Self-doubt is a real thing out here and I thank God I can overcome that every day. Thank you, God, for bringing and guiding me this far. I love you forever and I will never forget to point all my success back to you.

● ● ● ● ● ●

## 1/16/17

**T.G.I.M.** – Thank God It's Monday, I am so happy to be alive and healthy and able to do what I love. So today I had a good day in Modern class. I am really good at the "Flat back series."

I also enjoy doing Jason's "access the floor" passes. They feel very natural for me. In Meisha's class she gave me a couple of shoutouts because she saw me in ballet yesterday. I believe she appreciates my hard work and I know that is going to go a long way in my favor. At the end she taught a new combo. I ran it with every group because she said something about being the hardest worker in the room, including all your classes. That stuck with me so from now on I WILL be the hardest working in ALL my classes.

●  ●  ●  ●  ●  ●

# 5/17/2018

**Different Light** – The time I saw myself in a different light was when I performed in the cafe series and did a spoken word piece. I am usually only seen as a dancer, so this was a tad bit different. I remember feeling nerves that I never felt before. Not only was this my first time reciting spoken word on stage, with a mic, these were my words. I was completely vulnerable in a way I'd never been before. One of my friends recorded me and I remember just saying to myself, "Wow, this is me too." I realized I'm not just one thing; I am many things in one and my gifts, talents and creativity hold no limits.

# CHAPTER EIGHT
# A LINE TO HEAVEN

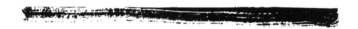

I put together a few prayers that are directly based from scripture. I use these prayers to guide me through repentance, shame, grief, pain, frustration and fear. I pray that these specific prayers will be the weapons of warfare that you put into practice in the rough seasons of your life as well as when you continue to step towards the greatest version of yourself.

● ● ● ● ● ●

## PRAYER FOR DIVINE MIGHT AND POWER

"And I pray that He would unveil within you the unlimited riches of His glory and favor until supernatural strength floods your innermost being with His divine might and explosive power."
– *Ephesians 3:16, TPT*

# PETITION PRAYER: PSALM 38, NIV
## A psalm of David. A petition.

LORD, do not rebuke me in your anger
    or discipline me in your wrath.
Your arrows have pierced me,
    and your hand has come down on me.
Because of your wrath there is no health in my body;
    there is no soundness in my bones because of my sin.
My guilt has overwhelmed me
    like a burden too heavy to bear.
My wounds fester and are loathsome
       because of my sinful folly.
I am bowed down and brought very low;
       all day long I go about mourning.
My back is filled with searing pain;
       there is no health in my body.
I am feeble and utterly crushed;
       I groan in anguish of heart.
All my longings lie open before you, Lord;
       my sighing is not hidden from you.
My heart pounds, my strength fails me;
       even the light has gone from my eyes.
My friends and companions avoid me because of my wounds;
       my neighbors stay far away.
Those who want to kill me set their traps,
       those who would harm me talk of my ruin;
       all day long they scheme and lie.

I am like the deaf, who cannot hear,
　　like the mute, who cannot speak;
I have become like one who does not hear,
　　whose mouth can offer no reply.
LORD, I wait for you;
　　you will answer, Lord my God.
For I said, "Do not let them gloat
　　or exalt themselves over me when my feet slip."
For I am about to fall,
　　and my pain is ever with me.
I confess my iniquity;
　　I am troubled by my sin.
Many have become my enemies without cause;
　　those who hate me without reason are numerous.
Those who repay my good with evil
　　lodge accusations against me,
　　though I seek only to do what is good.
LORD, do not forsake me;
　　do not be far from me, my God.
Come quickly to help me,
　　my Lord and my savior.

● ● ● ● ● ●

# PSALM 39, NIV
### For the director of music.
### For Jeduthun. A psalm of David.

I said, "I will watch my ways
     and keep my tongue from sin;
I will put a muzzle on my mouth
     while in the presence of the wicked."
So I remained utterly silent,
     not even saying anything good.
But my anguish increased;
  my heart grew hot within me.
While I meditated, the fire burned;
     then I spoke with my tongue:
"Show me, Lord, my life's end
     and the number of my days;
     let me know how fleeting my life is.
You have made my days a mere handbreadth;
     the span of my years is as nothing before you.
Everyone is but a breath,
     even those who seem secure.
"Surely everyone goes around like a mere phantom;
     in vain they rush about, heaping up wealth
     without knowing whose it will finally be.

"But now, Lord, what do I look for?
　　My hope is in you.
Save me from all my transgressions;
　　do not make me the scorn of fools.
I was silent; I would not open my mouth,
　　for you are the one who has done this.
Remove your scourge from me;
　　I am overcome by the blow of your hand.
When you rebuke and discipline anyone for their sin,
　　you consume their wealth like a moth—
　　surely everyone is but a breath.
"Hear my prayer, LORD,
　　listen to my cry for help;
　　do not be deaf to my weeping.
I dwell with you as a foreigner,
　　a stranger, as all my ancestors were.
Look away from me, that I may enjoy life again
　　before I depart and am no more."

# ROMANS 8, NIV

Therefore, there is now no condemnation for those who are in Christ Jesus, because through Christ Jesus the law of the Spirit who gives life has set you free from the law of sin and death. For what the law was powerless to do because it was weakened by the flesh, God did by sending his own Son in the likeness of sinful flesh to be a sin offering. And so he condemned sin in the flesh, in order that the righteous requirement of the law might be fully met in us, who do not live according to the flesh but according to the Spirit.

Those who live according to the flesh have their minds set on what the flesh desires; but those who live in accordance with the Spirit have their minds set on what the Spirit desires. The mind governed by the flesh is death, but the mind governed by the Spirit is life and peace. The mind governed by the flesh is hostile to God; it does not submit to God's law, nor can it do so. Those who are in the realm of the flesh cannot please God.

You, however, are not in the realm of the flesh but are in the realm of the Spirit, if indeed the Spirit of God lives in you. And if anyone does not have the Spirit of Christ, they do not belong to Christ. But if Christ is in you, then even though your body is subject to death because of sin, the Spirit gives life because of righteousness. And if the Spirit of him who raised Jesus from the dead is living in you, he who raised Christ from the dead will also give life to your mortal bodies because of his Spirit who lives in you.

Therefore, brothers and sisters, we have an obligation—but it is not to the flesh, to live according to it. For if you live according to the flesh, you will die; but if by the Spirit you put to death the misdeeds of the body, you will live.

For those who are led by the Spirit of God are the children of God. The Spirit you received does not make you slaves, so that you live in fear again; rather, the Spirit you received brought about your adoption to sonship. And by him we cry, "Abba, Father." The Spirit himself testifies with our spirit that we are God's children. Now if we are children, then we are heirs—heirs of God and co-heirs with Christ, if indeed we share in his sufferings in order that we may also share in His glory.

I consider that our present sufferings are not worth comparing with the glory that will be revealed in us. For the creation waits in eager expectation for the children of God to be revealed. For the creation was subjected to frustration, not by its own choice, but by the will of the one who subjected it, in hope that the creation itself will be liberated from its bondage to decay and brought into the freedom and glory of the children of God.

We know that the whole creation has been groaning as in the pains of childbirth right up to the present time. Not only so, but we ourselves, who have the first fruits of the Spirit, groan inwardly as we wait eagerly for our adoption to sonship, the redemption of our bodies. For in this hope we were saved. But hope that is seen is no hope at all. Who hopes for what they already have? But if we hope for what we do not yet have, we wait for it patiently.

In the same way, the Spirit helps us in our weakness. We do not know what we ought to pray for, but the Spirit himself intercedes for us through wordless groans. And he who searches our hearts knows the mind of the Spirit, because the Spirit intercedes for God's people in accordance with the will of God.

And we know that in all things God works for the good of those who love him, who have been called according to his purpose. For those God foreknew he also predestined to be conformed to the image of his Son, that he might be the firstborn among many brothers and sisters. And those he predestined, he also called; those he called, he also justified; those he justified, he also glorified.

What, then, shall we say in response to these things? If God is for us, who can be against us? He who did not spare his own Son, but gave him up for us all – how will he not also, along with him, graciously give us all things? Who will bring any charge against those whom God has chosen? It is God who justifies. Who then is the one who condemns? No one. Christ Jesus who died – more than that, who was raised to life—is at the right hand of God and is also interceding for us. Who shall separate us from the love of Christ? Shall trouble or hardship or persecution or famine or nakedness or danger or sword?

As it is written:
"For your sake we face death all day long;
   we are considered as sheep to be slaughtered."

No, in all these things we are more than conquerors through him who loved us. For I am convinced that neither death nor life, neither angels nor demons, neither the present nor the future, nor any powers, neither height nor depth, nor anything else in all creation, will be able to separate us from the love of God that is in Christ Jesus our Lord.

● ● ● ● ● ●

# PRAYER AGAINST SHAME & CONDEMNATION

Heavenly Father, my guilt has overwhelmed me like a burden too heavy to bear. My wounds fester and are loathsome because of my sinful folly. I am bowed down and brought very low. All day long I go about mourning. All my longings lie open before you Oh Lord, my sighing is not hidden from you. I confess my iniquity and I am troubled by my sin; but I rejoice in your name and word for you have said, so now there is no condemnation for those who are in Christ Jesus. I pray O Lord that you do not forsake me, be not far from me, O my God come quickly to help me. I will watch my ways and keep my tongue from sin. Dear Lord, I now put all my hope in you, save me from all my transgressions and do not make me the scorn of fools. Thank you, Lord, for loving me when I was even too foolish to love myself and for saving me from sin and myself. I will no longer condemn myself for you do not condemn me. I love you Lord and will commit my heart and ways to you, provide me with strength and heart to remain faithful and committed unto you Lord in Jesus name.

# HOSEA — JOEL PRAYER (REPENTANCE)

Heavenly Father forgive me all my sins and receive me graciously, that I may offer the food of my lips. You will heal my waywardness and love me freely, for your anger has turned away from me. I will be like the dew to Israel; He will blossom like a Lily. Like a Cedar of Lebanon, he will send down his roots; his young shoots will grow. Your splendor will be like an olive tree, your fragrance like a Cedar of Lebanon. I will dwell again in his shade. In Jesus name, you said you are sending me grain, new wine and oil, enough to satisfy me fully. I will see the new fresh anointing of you and your spirit over and in my life. Never again will you make me an object of scorn to the nations. Surely you, the Lord, has done and will continue to do great things. My open pastures are becoming green with your spirit. My trees are bearing fruit and the fig tree, and the vine yield their riches. I will rejoice and praise you Lord God for you send abundant showers and the threshing floors will be filled with grain, the vats will overflow with new wine and oil. In Jesus' name you said you will repay me for the years the locusts have eaten. I reclaim and you restore me from all past hurt, wickedness and damage the enemy has caused in my life, and I reverse all curses and brokenness, in the name of Jesus! Lord, reveal all brokenness in my life and hear me from the inside out. Thank you, Lord, for you have given me plenty to eat, until I am full, and I will praise your name Lord God. Never again will I be ashamed, for I know you are the Lord my God and that there is no other. Never again will I be shamed, in Jesus' precious name, AMEN!

# DARK ALLEY PRAYER

I will walk boldly under the Kingdom of Heaven, for Jesus holds my hand day and night with strength and might, that I may walk out the purpose and plan for my life courageously. Even through the mist of my enemies and being surrounded by darkness, the light of the Lord within me will be my saving grace and everlasting God. In the name of Jesus, Amen!

God leads me and guides my footsteps and my tongue so that I know exactly what to say and to whom. Bring people in need into my path so that your spirit leaves means of fellowship with them. I have no fear, for you are with me, and so your guardian angels forever are encamped around me. I ask you to genuinely press through and use me so that the Holy Spirit take me over to impact and touch the lives of everyone, especially the people who need it the most.

# AFTERWORD

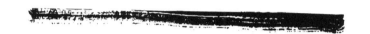

This is my life so far – my struggles, my pain, my plight – and if seeing my battle encourages you to fight, then I know I did right.

This is the end of this book and the beginning of my journey. Letting go of the past twenty years has been hard. I cried writing this book, I laughed remembering those times of joy, and I've been more vulnerable writing these words than I've ever been in my life. As I sit here writing these final thoughts, I can't help but zoom out of the microscope on my life and look at the bigger picture. I can't help but wonder if the world 100 years after I'm gone will be affected by what I've done in it. Will the angels of Heaven rejoice when I come home? Will my Father be proud of me? I think if I could leave you with a few things, it would be these:

## 1. You Are Who God Says You Are

- No matter what circumstance you've been through, the hand in life you were dealt, or the choices you've made, YOU ARE GREATNESS personified. You are beautiful and you have access to a Father in Heaven who will show you boundless love and an abundance of life, if you let him. You are royalty and you have authority over any and every plan and attack of the enemy. Believe you are who God says you are, and your life WILL be GREAT!

## 2. Vulnerability is Power

- The society and culture of the world today have tricked us into thinking that being open and vulnerable are signs of weakness; it's all a lie. Many of us, including myself, have experienced things in our lives that have ruined and tainted our ability to feel and our ability to be vulnerable with anybody, and especially with ourselves. It is even sometimes hard to be real and honest with ourselves because of what others have tricked us into believing. I want to tell you now that your vulnerability is powerful. Let me explain why. The power of life and death lies within your mouth and your words. Being vulnerable and speaking your truth does only one thing: bring life to a dead or dying situations in other people's lives. By you standing up and being vulnerable, your life has just become the key to unlocking the door of freedom, liberation and strength in another. All it takes is one person to live out the strength of vulnerability to liberate an entire generation. Will that one person be you?

## 3. Your Truth is YOUR TRUTH

- Never forget the vastness, the intensity and the weight of your truth. Do not let others diminish what you know to be true. I say this because oftentimes when we try to live out our truth it is downplayed, and sometimes disrespected. But no matter the response, your truth is YOUR truth. You must be brave enough to stand in it, and most importantly, share it. Remember all that the truth has shown you, what it has taught you, the good, bad and the ugly. Remember it all. It can be the fuel that lights the fire of a person who will go on to change the world, naturally and eternally.

I wrote this book to make it as personal as possible. If you know me then you know I only like to operate in extreme authenticity. I am writing these closing thoughts just as if you are here in this room with me, breathing the same air I am, almost perspiring because of how warm it is in here. I wrote this book and included my journal entries so you can get an overall sense of Jahred Rice, not the dancer, not the writer, not the goofy guy who always says everything is great; but Jahred Rice, the person. I've shared my life with you in the hope of encouraging you to take your next step to greatness. I've been open with you for you to be open with yourself, but also to the people who love and care about you.

To the people who feel like nobody cares or loves you, I can confidently say that is an absolute falsehood you should no longer choose to accept. First and foremost, God loves you past anything and everything you've experienced. He formed you and knew you before you were even born, and His love is unwavering. Secondly, whether I know you personally or not, whether you like me or not, or you have wronged me or vice versa: I LOVE YOU. This isn't me being cheesy and just saying it to sound good. I genuinely mean it and care for you. You are special. You are beautiful. You are great!

Thank you for reading this book, I pray your life has been changed because of it. Never forget to always live your truth, because the truth about the truth is it's yours, and only YOU can use it to change the world.

Made in the USA
Columbia, SC
08 July 2021